Thrive with Fibro

Delicious Eats for Energy & Relief

Jasmine Scott

Table Of Contents

Introduction

Do you crave delicious food but struggle with the fatigue and pain of fibromyalgia? You're not alone. Millions navigate this condition, and finding ways to manage symptoms while still enjoying life is key. "Thrive with Fibro: Delicious Eats for Energy & Relief" is your guide to a vibrant future fueled by both flavor and function.

This book isn't just a recipe collection; it's a roadmap to feeling your best. We'll explore how the right foods can become powerful allies in managing your fibromyalgia. From energizing breakfasts to feel-good comfort meals, we'll equip you with the knowledge and recipes to create a food lifestyle that supports your well-being. We won't forget the sweet tooth, either, with healthy dessert options that satisfy cravings without compromising your health goals.

Get ready to discover delicious dishes that nourish your body and soul. Let's embark on this journey together, one delicious bite at a time!

Chapter 1: Fibro Fighters: Food for Energy

Fibromyalgia. The word alone may cause a wave of tiredness, muscular pains, and sleep difficulties. This chronic ailment, which affects millions of people, predominantly women, has a negative impact on your energy and general health. But here's some good news: you're not powerless. While there is no cure, controlling your food may be an effective strategy in treating fibromyalgia and recovering your life.

This chapter delves into understanding fibromyalgia and how the appropriate meals may help you battle for energy and comfort.

Understanding Fibromyalgia

Fibromyalgia is a complicated disorder that produces widespread pain, discomfort, exhaustion, and sleep disturbances. Unlike injuries with an obvious cause, fibromyalgia pain seems to stem from faulty processing in the brain and spinal cord, which amplifies pain signals. This may have a domino effect, changing sleep habits, leaving you exhausted, and affecting your mood.

The Food and Fibromyalgia Connection
While the specific origin of fibromyalgia remains unknown, evidence indicates a substantial correlation between food and symptom management. Here's how food may contribute positively:

- Inflammation Fighters: Fibromyalgia is considered to be caused by chronic inflammation. Certain diets, especially those high in processed carbohydrates, bad fats, and gluten, may exacerbate inflammation. In contrast, an anti-inflammatory diet rich in fruits, vegetables, whole grains, and healthy fats might help lower inflammation and perhaps relieve pain.
- Energy Boosters: Many people with fibromyalgia suffer from fatigue on a daily basis. The correct nutrients may deliver consistent energy throughout the day. Complex carbs, which are found in healthy grains, fruits, and vegetables,

release energy gradually, eliminating the crashes that come with sugary foods.

- Sleep promoters: Fibromyalgia patients face significant challenges due to sleep disruptions. Some meals include chemicals that promote calm and improved sleep. Consider cherries, which are high in melatonin, or warm milk with a hint of turmeric, which is renowned for its relaxing benefits.
- Gut Health: Maintaining a healthy gut flora is critical to overall health. Some studies indicate a relationship between intestinal health and fibromyalgia symptoms. Including prebiotics and probiotics in your diet may help support the beneficial gut flora, perhaps improving symptoms.

Building Your Food Arsenal

Now that you understand the power of food, let's create your own "fibro fighter" arsenal. Here are some important dietary strategies:

- Embrace the Mediterranean Diet: This heart-healthy eating plan, which includes fruits, vegetables, whole grains, legumes, and healthy fats like olive oil, is a natural anti-inflammatory powerhouse.
- Remember Your Macros: Maintain a balanced macronutrient intake, including carbs, protein, and healthy fats. This provides continuous energy and keeps you feeling fuller for longer.
- Hydrate Right: Dehydration may aggravate tiredness in fibromyalgia patients. Aim for eight glasses of water each day, including hydrating fruits and vegetables such as watermelon and cucumber.
- Identify Food Triggers: Some persons with fibromyalgia discover that particular foods exacerbate their symptoms. Pay attention to how you feel after eating certain foods, such as gluten, dairy, or artificial sweeteners. Consider maintaining a food diary to monitor possible triggers.
- Read food labels. Be aware of hidden sugars, bad fats, and additives that might

cause inflammation. Learn to read food labels and choose whole, unprocessed foods wherever feasible.

Take the First Bite

Remember that implementing a new nutritional strategy is a journey, not a destination. Begin gradually, maybe by integrating one or two anti-inflammatory items into your regular diet. Experiment with the recipes in this book to experience the delight of delectable meals that nourish your body and combat exhaustion. Making intelligent food choices will help you manage your fibromyalgia and recapture your energy for a more vibrant life.

Chapter 2: Kitchen Staples: Easy Eats

Living with fibromyalgia may make even basic chores seem daunting. Cooking should not be another obstacle. This chapter is a refuge for cupboard and fridge essentials that may be transformed into fast, tasty, and nutritious meals. We'll concentrate on items that have a lengthy shelf life or may be prepared ahead of time, sparing you valuable energy.

Protein Powerhouses:

- Canned or pouched tuna/salmon: These adaptable fish are high in lean protein, omega-3 fatty acids, and vitamin D, all of which help to manage inflammation and weariness. Stock a variety for fast lunches and quick supper ideas.
- Frozen Skinless, Boneless Chicken Breasts: These freezer mainstays thaw fast and may be grilled, roasted, or pan-fried to provide a range of protein requirements. Marinate them ahead of time to get more flavor with less work.

- Lentils & Beans: These legumes are a vegetarian or vegan protein powerhouse, providing fiber, protein, and other minerals. Pre-cook a big quantity over the weekend and parcel it out for quick use in salads, soups, or stir-fries.
- Eggs: A complete protein with several applications, eggs are ideal for quick breakfasts, light meals, and protein boosts throughout the day. Hard-boiled eggs are a convenient snack, but scrambled eggs may be prepared in minutes.

Fiber Fantastic Friends:

- Frozen fruits and vegetables: Stock your freezer with these time-saving items. Frozen choices maintain the majority of their nutrients and are accessible all year round. They may be blended, stir-fried, or used as a soup basis.
- Canned beans and lentils (rinsed): They provide the same advantages as dry beans but do not need soaking. They're ideal for fast salads, dips, and

incorporating protein and fiber into soups and stews.

- Brown rice or quinoa: Whole grains are high in fiber and complex carbs, which provide long-lasting energy to help with tiredness management. Cook a big amount at the start of the week to simplify meal planning.
- Sweet potatoes are a nutritious and versatile vegetable. Roast them for a fast side dish, mash them for a creamy comfort meal, or substitute them for regular potatoes in recipes.

Healthy Fat Heroes:

- Olive Oil: This heart-healthy oil is essential for every kitchen. It may be used to make salad dressings, spreading over vegetables, or cooked at low heat.
- Avocado: This creamy fruit provides healthful fats and a hint of richness to salads, sandwiches, and smoothies.
- Nuts and seeds: Keep a variety of nuts and seeds on hand for snacking or to add nutritious crunch to salads, yogurt

parfaits, and stir-fries. They are high in healthy fats, protein, and fiber. To keep sodium consumption under control, choose unsalted kinds.

Flavor boosters:

- Herbs & spices: These pantry mainstays bring flavor and liveliness to every recipe, enabling you to experiment with novel flavor combinations without exerting too much effort. Experiment with fresh or dried herbs and spices to create unlimited combinations.
- Garlic and ginger: These potent components not only contribute flavor, but also have anti-inflammatory qualities. Store them fresh or frozen for quick access.
- Lemon and lime: Squeezing citrus enhances tastes and lends a refreshing touch to both savory and sweet recipes. They also assist to maintain the color of cut fruits and vegetables.

Pantry helpers:

- Canned tomatoes, whether crushed, diced, or whole, serve as a flexible basis for a variety of foods such as soups, sauces, and pasta.
- Chicken or vegetable broths give flavorful depth to soups, stews, and sauces. To keep your salt consumption under control, use low-sodium alternatives.
- Coconut milk is a creamy, non-dairy alternative that adds richness to curries, soups and smoothies.

Bonus tip: Batch cooking.

Batch cooking saves you even more time and energy. Choose a day to prepare a large amount of soup, stew, or protein, such as grilled chicken breasts. Portion them into containers for quick grab-and-go lunches all week.

Remember, your kitchen does not need to be a fight. This list provides a starting point for stocking your pantry and fridge so you can prepare tasty and healthy meals without sacrificing taste or convenience. Now, let's begin cooking!

Chapter 3: Mornings Made Easy: Power Breakfasts

The first meal of the day sets the tone for everything that follows. A well-designed breakfast is especially important for those with fibromyalgia. It gives an initial energy boost to get your day started and establishes the framework for controlling symptoms such as weariness and brain fog. But who has the stamina to prepare extravagant meals when simply getting out of bed is exhausting? Fear not, fellow warriors! This chapter focuses on quick, tasty, and strong breakfasts that will energize your body and mind without breaking a sweat.

Fueling for Energy:
Fibromyalgia impairs the body's normal energy generation. Breakfast provides an opportunity to restore exhausted resources and counteract weariness. Here's what to emphasize for a strong start:

- Complex carbohydrates give prolonged energy release, as opposed to simple sugars, which provide an initial rise followed by a collapse. Choose whole grains such as oatmeal, whole wheat bread, or barley.

- Protein keeps you feeling full and contains important amino acids for muscle building and repair. Greek yogurt, eggs, cottage cheese, and a handful of nuts and seeds are all excellent alternatives.
- Avocado, nut butter, and olive oil are all good sources of healthful fats. They delay digestion, keeping you full for longer and improving cognitive function.

Quick & Easy Champions:

The secret to a great morning routine is simplicity. Here are some champion dishes that need minimum preparation yet provide a powerful energy punch:

- Overnight oats: This takes little work the night before. Simply mix rolled oats, yogurt, milk (dairy or non-dairy), and a drizzle of honey or maple syrup in a jar. To add flavor and texture in the morning, top with fresh berries, nuts, or a dab of nut butter.

- Power Smoothie Bowl: This breakfast is both gorgeous and tasty. Blend together frozen fruit (berries, banana, mango), a scoop of protein powder, spinach or kale, and your preferred milk. Pour into a bowl and garnish with granola, chia seeds, and a dollop of Greek yogurt.
- Scrambled Eggs with Spinach and Feta: In less than 10 minutes, you can prepare this protein-packed dish. Sauté some chopped spinach in olive oil, then scramble a few eggs with crumbled feta cheese. Season with salt and pepper and serve on whole wheat bread.

Make-ahead Magic:

On those mornings when exhaustion sets in, planning ahead of time comes in handy. Here are some make-ahead suggestions for a stress-free morning routine:

- Hard-boiled Eggs: On the weekend, boil a batch of eggs to keep on hand throughout the week. They're packed with protein and healthy fats, making them ideal for a fast grab-and-go meal.

- Chia Pudding: Soak chia seeds in your chosen milk with a splash of sugar overnight. In the morning, garnish with fresh fruit, nuts, or granola.
- Baked Oatmeal Cups: Divide your favorite oatmeal recipe into muffin cups and bake ahead of time. These may be reheated in the microwave for a warm, filling breakfast.

Don't Forget Hydration.

Hydration is essential for controlling fibromyalgia symptoms, particularly exhaustion and cognitive fog. Make water your first beverage of the day. If plain water is too bland, add slices of cucumber, lemon, or berries for taste. Herbal teas are another great alternative, with added advantages such as enhanced gut health and relaxation.

Embrace the power of batch cooking.

If you have time on weekends, try preparing some breakfast components ahead of time. Chop your veggies, make a bowl of brown rice, or measure out nuts and seeds. Having these ingredients on hand simplifies preparing a nutritious breakfast.

Listen to your body.
Remember that there is no one-size-fits-all approach to breakfast. Experiment to see what works best for you. Some days, you may need a warm and soothing cup of oatmeal, while others may require a speedy protein shake. Pay attention to your body's messages and adapt your decisions appropriately.

Embrace variety.
While consistency is beneficial, keep things interesting by include variation in your breakfast options. Experiment with various fruits, veggies, and spices to keep your palate satisfied and motivated.

With a little forethought and these tasty breakfast options, you can conquer your mornings and feel motivated to face the day ahead. Remember that a simple investment in a nutritious breakfast may go a long way toward fuelling your body and reducing fibromyalgia symptoms. Now, go out and conquer your day, one tasty piece at a time!

Chapter 4: Comfort & Relief: Feel-Good Food

Fibromyalgia might cause days when all you want is a warm embrace in a bowl. This chapter explores the world of comfort food, but with a healthier twist! We'll look at dishes that are not only tasty and gratifying, but also include anti-inflammatory substances to help you control your symptoms and boost overall well-being.

These are not your typical calorie-laden comfort meals. We'll concentrate on nutrients high in omega-3 fatty acids, antioxidants, and gut-friendly bacteria, all of which have been shown to help reduce inflammation and promote a healthy gut flora, which may have a substantial influence on fibromyalgia symptoms.

Let's have a look at some delicious foods that can calm both your body and spirit.

1. Creamy Turmeric Chicken Stew: This recipe is the epitome of comfort.

Turmeric, a potent anti-inflammatory spice, takes center stage, adding warmth and earthy flavor to the recipe. Chicken offers lean protein, while vegetables such as carrots, celery, and potatoes provide vitamins and fiber. Coconut milk provides a creamy, soothing foundation, while ginger adds a hint of zest.

2. Salmon with Roasted Vegetables and Lemon Dill Sauce: Salmon is rich in omega-3 fatty acids, which have anti-inflammatory qualities. Roasting veggies such as broccoli, asparagus, and cherry tomatoes enhances their natural sweetness, while a simple lemon dill sauce gives a burst of freshness. This recipe is not only tasty, but also visually stunning, making it ideal for a cozy and gratifying supper.

3. Lentil Soup with Whole-Wheat Bread: Humble lentils are high in protein and fiber, making them an ideal basis for a substantial and healthy soup. They also possess anti-inflammatory effects. This

soup is made using vegetables such as carrots, onions, and celery, resulting in a thick and savory broth. Toasted whole-wheat bread gives a pleasant texture while also providing complex carbs for lasting energy.

4. Chicken and Vegetable Stir-fry with Brown Rice: Stir-fries are an excellent method to prepare a fast and nutritious supper. This dish includes lean chicken breast and a variety of bright veggies such as bell peppers, broccoli florets, and snow peas. The stir-fry is served with a light sauce prepared with low-sodium soy sauce, ginger, garlic, and a touch of honey for a savory and slightly sweet taste profile. Brown rice has a nutty taste and contains complex carbs that give long-lasting energy.

5. Anti-Inflammatory Smoothie Bowl: Smoothies are an easy and tasty method to get a lot of nutrients. This dish includes antioxidant-rich fruits such as berries and mango, which may help reduce

inflammation. Spinach gives a hidden dose of greens, while a scoop of protein powder provides necessary building blocks for muscle repair. Granola, chia seeds, and chopped almonds provide texture and healthy fats to a breakfast or snack bowl, making it both filling and visually attractive.

Remember, these are only beginning points! Feel free to experiment with various ingredients and flavors to make recipes that fit your tastes.

Tips for Comforting Touches:

1. Fresh Herbs: A sprinkling of fresh herbs, such as parsley, cilantro, or dill, may quickly brighten and refresh any meal.
2. Spice it Up: Do not be scared to experiment with spices! Ginger, garlic, turmeric, and cayenne pepper not only enhance taste but also have anti-inflammatory qualities.
3. Healthy Fats: Include avocado, olive oil, and nuts in your meals. These fats not

only increase satiety, but also help to reduce inflammation.

4. Bone Broth: Making a pot of bone broth is an excellent method to provide a nutritious basis for soups and stews. Bone broth is high in collagen, which helps promote joint health.

By combining these suggestions and dishes into your diet, you can create a world of comfort food that not only calms your spirit but also improves your overall health while you navigate your fibromyalgia journey. Remember, food is powerful; utilize it to your advantage!

Chapter 5: Sweet Indulgences: Healthier Treats Satisfying cravings

Living with fibromyalgia might seem like an ongoing fight. You control your discomfort, battle weariness, and prioritize your health. But what about those occasions when a sweet treat calls your name? Can you enjoy without jeopardizing your health goals? Absolutely! This chapter is a paradise for delectable, delightful treats that will not make you feel guilty or worse.

We all want sweets from time to time. It may be a mood enhancer, a pick-me-up after a hard day, or just a way to round off a meal on a positive note. The trick is to identify healthier options that meet your desires without including processed sweets, bad fats, or inflammatory substances.

This chapter reveals a treasure trove of delectable delicacies, which include

- Lower in Sugar: We'll utilize natural sweeteners like dates, maple syrup, and even ripe fruits to provide sweetness without the blood sugar rise caused by processed sugars.

- Packed with Nutrients: Many of these dishes include nuts, seeds, and whole grains, which provide healthy fats, fiber, and critical vitamins and minerals.
- Anti-Inflammatory Powerhouses: We'll look at nutrients having anti-inflammatory characteristics, such as berries, dark chocolate, and some spices, that may benefit your general health.

Here are some culinary ideas that will make your taste buds tingle.

- Fruity Bliss Balls: These no-bake snacks are full of flavor and texture. Dates serve as the basis, which is combined with nut butter, rolled oats, and a variety of chopped fruits such as dried cranberries, blueberries, and apples. A sprinkling of chia seeds provides a lovely crunch.

- Creamy Avocado Mousse: Despite its decadence, this mousse is really rather nutritious. Avocados provide a thick, creamy texture, while cocoa powder and a splash of maple syrup provide a delightful chocolaty flavor. Consider adding a sprinkle of espresso powder or a teaspoon of vanilla essence to enhance the taste.

- Baked Apples with Spiced Nuts: A traditional comfort dish gets a healthier twist. Core apples and fill with a combination of chopped nuts such as walnuts and pecans, drizzled with honey, and topped with warming spices like as cinnamon, nutmeg, and ginger. Bake until the apples are soft and the filling aromatic. Add a dollop of Greek yogurt or whipped coconut cream for a luscious finish.

- Chia Seed Pudding with Berries: This overnight wonder is ideal for hectic mornings or a filling afternoon snack. Mix chia seeds with your favorite nut milk, a splash of maple syrup, and a teaspoon of vanilla essence. Let it set in the fridge overnight, then top with fresh berries in the morning.

- Healthy Brownies: You will not believe how amazing these brownies are for you! These brownies, made with whole wheat flour, mashed banana for sweetness, and natural cocoa powder, are high in fiber and taste. Add a handful of chopped dark chocolate pieces for added enjoyment (and antioxidants!).

Remember, these are merely starting points for your creativity. Experiment with various taste combinations and healthful components to find your unique preferences. Here are some more guidelines for managing the world of sweets with fibromyalgia:

- Portion Control: Even healthful foods should be consumed in moderation. Use smaller dishes or ramekins to limit portion sizes and avoid overeating.
- Mindful Eating: Enjoy each mouthful, paying attention to the flavor and texture.

This helps you to savor the dessert more and maybe be happy with a lesser piece.

- Pair with Protein: When eating a sweet treat, try matching it with a protein source, such as a handful of almonds or a dollop of Greek yogurt. This helps manage blood sugar levels and keeps you feeling fuller for longer.
- Listen to your body. Pay attention to how you feel after you indulge. If a certain dessert causes discomfort or weariness, take note and select a different alternative the next time.

Living with fibromyalgia does not exclude enjoying sweet sweets. With a little imagination and these nutritious dishes, you can fulfill your appetites while putting your health first. So go ahead, eat guilt-free, and enjoy the delightful route to a healthy you!

Conclusion

Congratulations! You've completed "Thrive with Fibro: Delicious Eats for Energy & Relief." We hope this book has inspired you to adopt a culinary habit that promotes your health and ignites your battle against fibromyalgia. Remember that food is a strong instrument. You can nourish your body, improve your energy, and feel more vital by making smart decisions and adopting these tasty dishes.

This trip does not finish here. Continue to experiment with different dishes and tastes, and learn how food might help you manage your fibromyalgia symptoms. Most importantly, recognize your accomplishments, large and little. Every nutritious meal you pick is a step towards a better future.

We wish you ongoing strength, perseverance, and a plate full of great options!